Don't Just
STAND THERE

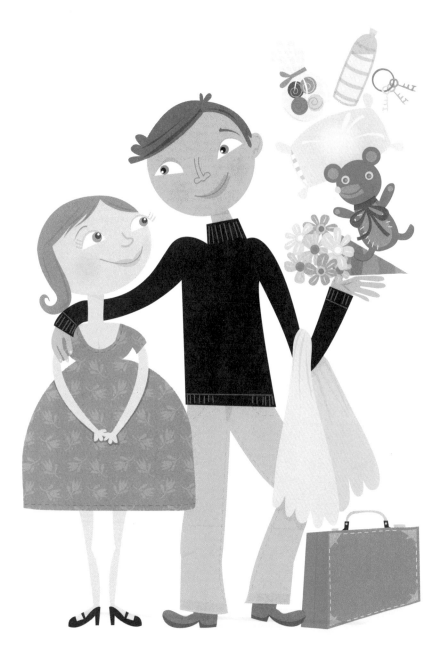

Don't Just
STAND THERE

How to Be Helpful, Clued-In, Supportive, Engaged,
Meaningful, and Relevant in the Delivery Room

By Elissa Stein and Jon Lichtenstein
Illustrations by Beegee Tolpa

CHRONICLE BOOKS
SAN FRANCISCO

Library of Congress Cataloging-in-Publication Data:

Stein, Elissa.
    Don't just stand there : how to be helpful, clued-in, supportive, engaged,
    meaningful, and relevant in the delivery room /
by Elissa Stein and Jon Lichtenstein.
        p. cm.
    ISBN-13: 978-0-8118-5569-3
    ISBN-10: 0-8118-5569-4
    Includes bibliographical references and index.
1. Labor (Obstetrics)—Popular works. 2. Childbirth—Popular works.
3. Fathers—Attitudes—Popular works. I. Lichtenstein, Jon. II. Title.

    RG652.S694 2007
        618.4—dc22

                        2006012070

Manufactured in China.

Design by Danielle Foushée

Distributed in Canada by Raincoast Books
9050 Shaughnessy Street
Vancouver, British Columbia V6P 6E5

10 9 8 7 6 5 4 3 2 1

Chronicle Books LLC
680 Second Street
San Francisco, California 94107

www.chroniclebooks.com

Cheetos and Doritos are registered trademarks of Frito-Lay North America,
Inc. iPod is a registered trademark of Apple Computer, Inc. LifeSavers is
a registered trademark of Nabisco Brands, Inc. Monopoly is a registered
trademark of Hasbro Inc. Pitocin is a registered trademark of Warner-Lambert
Co. TiVo is a registered trademark of TiVo Brands LLC. Ziploc is a registered
trademark of S.C. Johnson Home Storage, Inc.

For Nomi, Sara, and Adam

CONTENTS

Forewords • 8

Introduction • 11

Stages of Labor • 15

What to Bring • 47

What to Say • 53

How to Comfort • 69

What Not to Do, Say, or Bring • 91

Fill in the Blanks • 95

Acknowledgments • 100

Resources • 101

Index • 103

FOREWORDS

"Nothing can truly prepare you for childbirth."

I find myself saying these words over and over again to expectant mothers and their partners in their last weeks of pregnancy. It's a time filled with tremendous anticipation and joy—and fear, as well. I tell expectant parents to read as much as they can; to talk to their mothers, sisters, and friends; and to do everything they can think of to prepare themselves. I firmly believe that when you're as prepared as you can be, the birthing experience will be much more positive for everyone.

To that end, *Don't Just Stand There* offers precise, practical tips that make a big difference in the delivery room. Rarely is the subject addressed, but labor can be very hard on the birthing partner. You may feel powerless, scared, and worried about the mom-to-be. This wonderful and informative book outlines everything you need to know to be helpful and understand what's happening as labor unfolds.

Don't Just Stand There will make you think about, prepare for, laugh at, and embrace what's about to happen. It's sure to help you and your partner get through the crazy process that we call *labor*.

- Dr. Suzanne LaJoie, MD, Downtown Women Ob-Gyn Associates, LLP, New York, NY

As you and your partner know by now, pregnancy is a time of rapid change. Along with her changing body come rapidly changing thoughts and emotions. A mom-to-be can hardly keep track of all these changes—let alone you, the future dad. When labor starts, changes happen even faster, and they're even more momentous: labor brings about not only the birth of the baby but also the birth of a new mother and father.

For many couples, playing an active, integral role in the birth experience is exactly the start to parenthood they are seeking. For others, just getting through labor as smoothly as possible is enough of a goal. Regardless of which perspective you have, this book offers, in a practical and playful format, great tips to help you through your childbirth experience. *Don't Just Stand There* will make you laugh, while giving you essential information.

Most important, amid all the wonderful tips and explanations offered here, you'll learn that the one thing your partner really needs while she is going through this life-changing experience is you. Not a single trick of the trade will help as much as knowing that you are there with her, 100 percent of the way. Just be present with her. Let her know that she is not alone and you love her. While everything is changing and the challenges seem to be never-ending, she will be comforted knowing you are by her side, loving her and willing to help.

In your inevitable moments of change and confusion, I hope this book and referring to it through your experience will provide the supportive companion that you need.

- Jessica Kramer, Doula & LMT, Los Angeles, CA

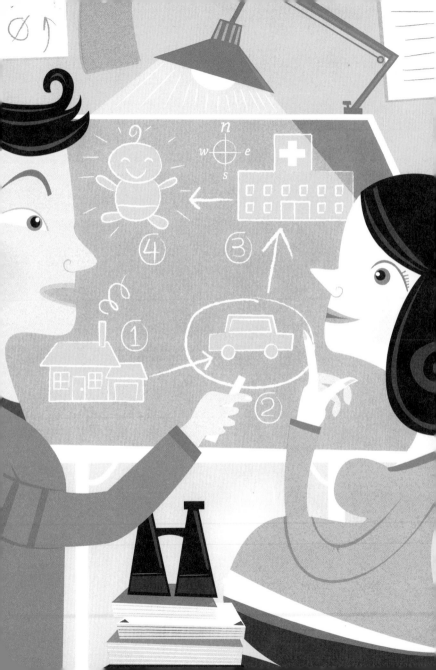

Childbirth is a free-for-all. No matter how much you and your partner plan, you can never truly be prepared for an event so unpredictable, unscheduled, and, quite frankly, uncomfortable. Even if you take the birthing classes, practice breathing techniques, and listen to your partner talk endlessly about books she's read telling her what to expect, when you are woken up at three in the morning or get that phone call pulling you out of a meeting, everything goes out the window. You're about to go through a life-changing experience, and you're likely to forget everything you've learned along the way.

She's going to be stressed and a little bit on edge. Someone's got to step up and ease the strain a bit. And that someone is you. Believe it or not, there's plenty that you can do to help the mom-to-be relax, or at least to be more comfortable in a very uncomfortable situation.

That's why this book came into being. After my first birth experience, which was confusing, chaotic, and completely unlike anything we had prepared for, I was determined to do as much as I could to have a better experience the second time around. We found a remarkable doula (a woman who provides support during labor) who made us both more comfortable and, believe it or not, actually helped us find humor and ease in the delivery room. I put together a handbook for my husband, Jon (the male voice you'll find throughout the book), to use while I was in labor—positive words I thought I'd want to hear, prompts for him to lead me through visualizations and deep breathing, and guidelines for him to follow (absolutely no picture-taking after a certain point; music selection was non-negotiable). It worked. Having him be more involved helped me, and it helped him by giving him things to do, ask, or suggest. He became a positive and involved player in the experience.

This book is designed to help you help your partner deal with the challenges of labor, both by guiding your planning (with space in back for you to fill in your own ideas, too) and by supplying plenty of suggestions for things to try during labor. Within these pages you'll find advice culled from moms, midwives, doulas, and ob-gyns—plus words of wisdom from an experienced dad—to help you two through.

And let's not forget about you. All of the focus is on the mom-to-be (and let's be honest, that's basically how it should be), but you're going through a fair amount of stress, exhaustion, and confusion yourself, so we've got stuff in here just for you.

The book is broken into sections that can be used for planning (should you be that organized) or for quick reference during labor.

Stages of Labor will walk you through—what else?—the stages of labor, outlining what to expect, and what you can do, during each stage. The chapter will help you keep track of things as labor progresses. Plus, you'll find questions to ask the professionals so you'll know exactly what stage she's at and what's going on. While hospital personnel deliver babies every day, you're new to child-birth, and knowing exactly what to ask can help cut through the confusion.

In **What to Bring,** you'll find a packing list of items that will help you both through labor and delivery. Before you read any further, stop and throw some deodorant and a toothbrush into your bag. Trust us, you'll need them by the time the baby arrives.

The **What to Say** chapter is full of affirmations, breathing prompts, and simple visualization ideas for you to read to her. Over and over if you need to. Over and over.

In **How to Comfort,** you'll find ideas for making her room feel cozier, tricks that can help ease tension, massage techniques (don't worry, nothing too complicated), and a guide to pressure points that can help with pain relief. Maybe these things will work for her, maybe not—you can never tell what will make a positive difference, so we have included as many options as possible for you to try out.

Then there's **What Not to Do, Say, or Bring.** Need we say more? We've included lots of suggestions here, but as a general rule, you'd do well to keep sports analogies to a minimum. She doesn't need to hear "you're near the end zone" more than once.

HE SAYS:

> I was asked to participate in this book on the strength of two factors: (1) my wife is the author, and (2) I was in the room both times she gave birth.

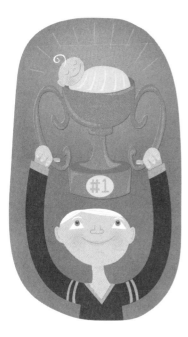

Okay, so I'm not an expert. But, long before my wife wrote this book, she wrote a book just for me, a mini *Don't Just Stand There*, which really gave me a central role in her second birth. Since I was the inspiration for this book, it made sense for me to throw in my two cents.

In chiming in, I will give you the "guy's perspective" to keep things honest and realistic. I promise, everything in here is appropriate for most guys. Don't worry—perineal massage is not on the recommended list.

So, why do you need this book? Nobody wants to feel like a third wheel, getting in the way. So whether you picked this book out for yourself (fat chance), or she gave it to you, it doesn't matter. You're going to be in the delivery room. And on that most incredible and memorable day of your life, you don't want to just stand there, do you?

Read on and pay attention. Being a great labor partner is merely the prelude to being a great dad.

Stages of
LABOR

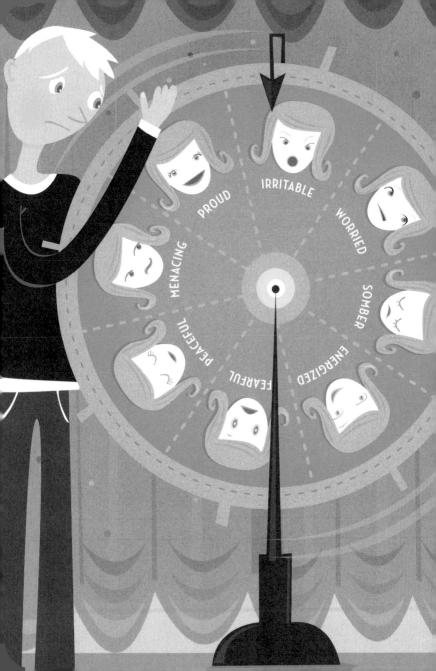

Every woman's labor is different. And each stage of labor brings new physical challenges, along with a range of emotions running the gamut from excitement to anticipation to fear.

But don't panic. There are several aspects of labor that you can count on regardless of the circumstances. Physically, a woman's body has to go through specific changes to prepare for the baby's birth. Knowing what to anticipate will help you to help her in the delivery room. That's what this section is all about. In the following pages, we've broken down labor into its major stages. And we've broken down each stage into three sections to explain what's going on with her physically, how she might be feeling emotionally, and what you can do to help.

We're going to walk you through what's likely to happen in the delivery room and tell you how to determine where she is in the labor process—and we've included lots of ideas about how you can help. Keep in mind that labor is unpredictable. Don't get caught up in what you *think* should be happening. Pay attention and respond to what *is* happening.

HE SAYS:

Labor is a wild ride. It will help both of you to know what gear she's in.

WHEN LABOR IS COMING SOON

Before labor starts, many moms-to-be show signs that it's coming, even if they don't recognize them as such. You may notice that your partner has a sudden urge to clean, or "nest"—organizing and getting things ready for the baby's arrival. (My mother scrubbed the kitchen floor on her hands and knees with a toothbrush right before she went into labor.) Or she may feel like sitting and watching videos for hours on end and not moving (my sign that labor was on its way). It could be that she feels something's not quite right, yet she can't pinpoint what it is. At this point, her body is preparing her for the job ahead, and she needs to reserve and store up energy for labor. So, should she have those energetic cleaning sprees, make sure she rests up afterward.

DUE DATES

A woman's due date is not the day she's likely to give birth. Actually, fewer than 5 percent of pregnant women give birth on their due date, which is 40 weeks from the first day of a woman's last period. A baby is considered full-term at any point from 38 to 42 weeks. So don't hang your hat on the due date, thinking it's a given—you never know.

HE SAYS:

Notwithstanding the odds, it's probably a good date to keep open.

What's happening to her body

- Her back may ache.

- She may need much more sleep than usual.

- There may be a dramatic change in her appetite.

- She may feel like she's under the weather.

- She could have occasional contractions, called Braxton Hicks contractions. These can occur throughout pregnancy, but they may increase in frequency as her due date gets closer. Unlike labor contractions, though, they do not grow consistently stronger, longer, and closer together.

What she's feeling

She could feel obsessive, exhausted, irritable, lethargic, cranky, energized, or anxious.

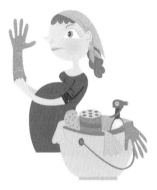

What you can do

- Be supportive. If she asks you to clean out the garage for the baby, don't question it.

- Indulge her sleeping needs. She's got hard work ahead of her.

- Make sure she stays hydrated and has plenty to eat.

You may not notice much at this stage. It's likely that, as she moved into the final trimester, you got used to her doing quirky things or complaining about aches and pains. So it's easy to write off signs that labor is approaching as just more of the same. In fact, you may miss this stage completely. Don't worry, once labor really starts, there's no missing it.

CESAREAN SECTIONS

Some women choose to have an elective Cesarean section, which is quite a different experience from going through labor. You pick a time and date (thus choosing your baby's birthday!), arrive at the hospital, and head to surgery, where the baby is surgically removed from the uterus. A C-section might also be necessary if the mother or baby gets into any sort of distress during labor. Either way, a Cesarean section is major surgery and will take time to recover from. Regardless of how the birth unfolds, and whether or not it went according to plan, a healthy mother and baby are the goal.

PRE-LABOR

There is nothing "pre" about pre-labor. For many women, pre-labor lasts for hours (and hours) and is punctuated by regular contractions that don't increase in intensity, length, or frequency. It's the stage of labor where everything you want to see happening is happening, but nothing appears to be progressing or changing. Being in this "holding pattern" can be emotionally taxing and exhausting. Try to keep the mom-to-be resting. She needs to conserve her energy. But if she feels like walking and moving around might help move things along, fine. Just make sure she gets lots of rest afterward.

What's happening to her body

- Contractions occur in an irregular pattern and may go on for days.

- She may lose her mucous plug, which has been sealing off her cervix. Losing the mucous plug, however, doesn't necessarily mean that labor is about to start.

HE SAYS:

> The mucous plug isn't like the plug in the bathtub. It's not holding her amniotic fluid in. I can't believe I thought that! Losing her mucous plug has nothing to do with her water breaking—that's something totally different (see page 24).

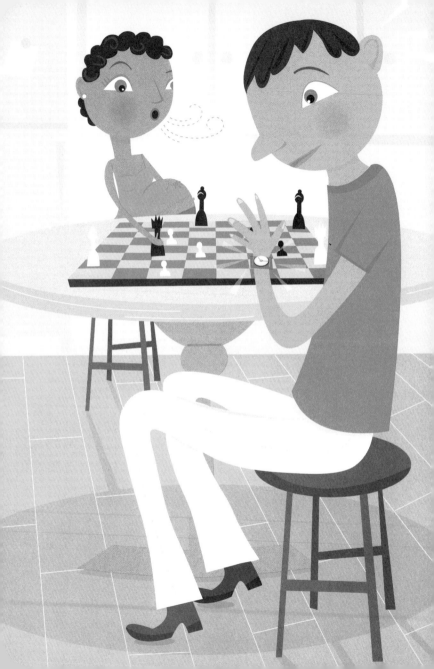

What she's feeling

Should pre-labor go on for a while, she'll probably feel really frustrated that labor hasn't "officially" started, or that no one is calling it labor when it sure feels like labor. She might also be tired, as contractions make it hard to get much rest. Or she might feel ready to go to the hospital, even though she's not dilating.

What you can do

- If pre-labor lasts for a while (it can go on for hours), make sure she gets plenty of rest and eats and drinks enough.

- Don't rush off to the hospital. If contractions aren't progressing, she won't be dilating yet and you will likely be sent back home. It can be awfully discouraging to make the journey to the hospital only to be told things have not progressed enough for her to be admitted.

- Be encouraging, supportive, and patient.

- Try to keep her entertained and thinking about something besides labor. Watch movies. Play board games. Find her a trashy novel to read.

HE SAYS:

Now is the time to double-check your hospital bag, to make sure you've got everything you think you'll both want or need (see page 47).

WATER BREAKING

Many people think that the water breaking signals the start of labor. Nope—that's not necessarily true. Her water could break at any time—before labor kicks in or during any stage of labor. It could be a huge gush or a slow trickle. If her water doesn't break on its own during labor, her medical team might decide to break it, which can cause labor to progress more rapidly. Why? Because amniotic fluid eases pressure on the cervix, and when the watery cushion is gone the baby presses more firmly on the cervix, signaling it to open up. If your partner's medical team is talking about breaking her water, discuss it first—there are risks involved. Don't think of it as just a way of speeding up labor. Once her water breaks, both she and the baby are more prone to infection and there will be pressure to deliver the baby within 24 hours. Intercourse is discouraged, as are baths (that is, if her water breaks before labor kicks in—if she's already laboring, a nice soak is fine).

HE SAYS:

Intercourse?!?! After her water breaks and soaks the entire bed, it's perfectly fine to tell her you're not in the mood.

If her water breaks and labor doesn't kick in, her medical team may advise inducing labor with the drug Pitocin. Ask if there are alternative ways to get labor started if you want to hold off on medication.

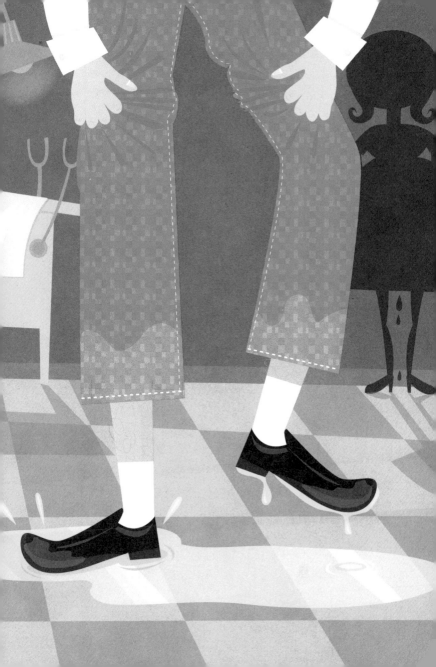

STAGE 1 LABOR

Stage 1 is all about contracting and dilating. Her uterus contracts with increasing regularity, and these intense muscle contractions help her cervix dilate (it will need to open up from 1 centimeter to 10 centimeters before she can start pushing), efface (get thinner, to allow the baby to pass through), and move the baby through the birth canal. Stage 1 has three distinct phases to it, generally determined by how dilated she is. A word of advice: Let go of time expectations—eventually all women get to Stage 2.

EARLY PHASE (STAGE 1)

This part of labor usually lasts a while. She'll most likely be more comfortable staying home for as long as possible during this phase—it's far better than sitting in traffic or being in a hospital waiting room. If you can't be home with her, make sure you're reachable and, if possible, that she has someone there to keep her company.

What's happening to her body

- Contractions occur with increasing regularity and frequency. They could be anywhere from 5 to 30 minutes apart.

- Her cervix dilates from 1 centimeter to 3 centimeters.

- Her back could hurt. At this stage, walking or moving around might make her feel more comfortable and assist with the progression of labor.

- She could experience nausea or diarrhea—all the activity in her abdomen can stir things up—which is perfectly normal.

What she's feeling

She might feel anxious, especially if she's a first-time mother.

What you can do

- Make sure she's drinking plenty of liquids.

- Have her eat high-energy snacks if she's willing—dried or fresh fruit, fruit juice (especially grape), and tea with honey are all terrific energy boosters. Stay away from citrus juices, though, which can irritate her stomach. If her labor is progressing slowly, encourage her to eat more substantial foods instead, like pasta, bagels, or peanut butter sandwiches.

- Help keep track of contractions—how long they last and how far apart they are. But don't get too obsessive—time a few and then take a break. A general rule: Before you go to the hospital, she should have eight to twelve consecutive contractions that last at least a minute each, are fewer than five minutes apart, and are intense enough that she needs to concentrate on getting through each one.

- Stay in touch with her doctor/midwife/doula and keep them posted about what's going on. Together you'll decide when the time is right to head to the birthing facility.

- Focus on her during contractions. This is not a good time for you to be multitasking (turn off the basketball game).

- Offer positive words of support and encouragement (see page 53).

HE SAYS:

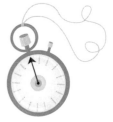

You may need to be the voice of reason here. She may be desperate to get to the hospital or birthing center, but don't let her push you out the door too quickly. You really want to make only one car trip with a laboring woman, if you can help it. Plus, it's much easier to be comfortable at home than in the hospital. So keep your wits and keep track of how long and how frequent those contractions are. This is probably a good time to confirm with yourself that you know how to get to the hospital and that there's gas in the car.

ACTIVE PHASE (STAGE 1)

As contractions become more frequent and intense, dilation progresses. This is when labor really kicks in.

What's happening to her body

- Contractions generally increase in frequency from every five minutes to every two to three minutes, and usually last from 30 to 60 seconds. They are much more regular now than in the early phase.

- Contractions become so intense that she can't talk through them anymore.

- Her cervix dilates from 4 centimeters to 7 centimeters.

What she's feeling

Her mood can fluctuate quickly as her body gets ready to give birth. Initial excitement often wanes as this phase gets progressively harder and more uncomfortable. Frustration could set in if dilation does not progress quickly.

What you can do

Now is the time to get her to the birthing facility. As labor is getting harder, it will help to settle in one place so she can get comfortable in her space and concentrate on labor, not on traffic or finding a cab.

This is the time to jump in and really help keep her focused and calm. Remember, if she just wants you to rub her back or hold her hand, go with it. Very often in this stage, one thing will work for her and it will become a ritual with each contraction. Try some of the following and see if anything clicks.

- Talk her through breathing prompts (see page 61).
- Read her a visualization or two (see page 63).
- Try some massage (see page 77).
- Work on acupressure points (see page 78).
- Make sure she's staying hydrated. Give her a sip of water after every contraction.
- Encourage her to rest between contractions. And if she yells at that suggestion, don't make it again.
- Walking can help here. If she feels comfortable being on her feet, let her hold on to you when a contraction hits.
- A warm shower might feel good at this point.
- Suggest different positions. Eventually she'll find something that feels just right.
- If she wants pain medication or an epidural, this is the time to talk to her medical team about administering the drugs.
- Continue giving her positive support and encouragement (see page 56).

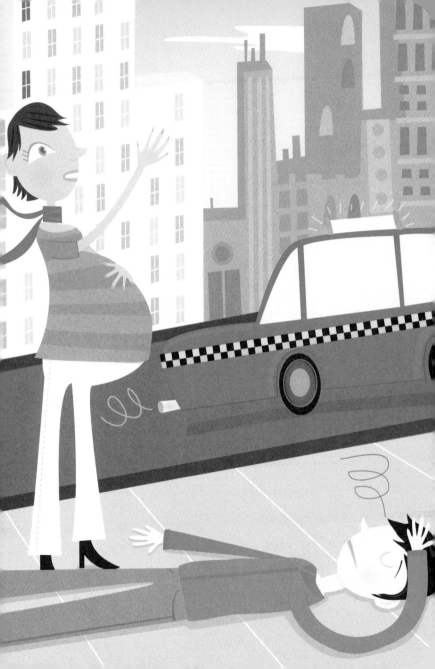

Okay, take a second and tell yourself you can do this. Just remember, you're a guy; you're tough. No matter how bad the pain gets, don't forget, you're not the one experiencing it.

TRANSITION (STAGE 1)

Transition is the point at which many women lose steam. She may say she wants to give up, go home—that she's changed her mind about having a baby. The transition phase is so intense because the body is making a major shift—it's finishing up dilating the cervix and switching gears to move the baby out of her body. The intensity of contractions can be terrifying and overwhelming—it's easy for her to lose sight of the fact that this won't last forever. The good news is that it will actually go by very quickly—the transition phase usually doesn't last more than an hour, or 25 contractions, and sometimes it takes just 2 or 3 contractions.

What's happening to her body

- Her cervix dilates from 8 centimeters to 10 centimeters.

- Contractions are incredibly intense now. They generally occur every two to three minutes and last for 60 seconds or more. Some contractions may follow one after another without any breaks in between.

- She might throw up, shake uncontrollably, and feel super-sensitive to touch.

- She will most likely feel very hot and be sweating.

What she's feeling

The transition is the most physically challenging and scary of the stages. She may panic and lose control. She may shake and shiver, doubt herself, and feel like a failure. She might also feel a strong urge to have a bowel movement. Most likely it's not a bowel movement; that's the baby.

HE SAYS:

Be calm. Be strong. Be supportive. She may curse you like a sailor. Under normal circumstances this might really make you laugh, but don't laugh now. Whatever foul names she's calling you, just keep agreeing with her. She needs to let it out and to keep breathing, so her body can do what it was designed to do.

What you can do

- Keep telling her it's only temporary, that this won't last forever.

- Remind her that her body can do this.

- Lock eyes with her and talk her through each contraction. Tell her to take it one breath at a time.

- Have her breathe with you, following your breath exactly—just one breath at a time.

- She may feel like she needs to push, but if she's not fully dilated, help her hold off.

- Help her focus on breathing instead of pushing by having her imagine she is blowing out a candle.

- Talk about how each contraction is bringing the baby closer.

- If she gets anxious or panicky, stay calm and softly talk her through it.

- When she's hot and sweaty, placing a cold washcloth on her forehead will make you a hero.

MEDICATION

Whether or not to use medication during childbirth is a personal choice. Keep in mind that it can be given only during certain points of labor. Should your partner have decided ahead of time that she wants an epidural, she generally needs to be 4 centimeters dilated before it will be administered. There are other pain medications available, which need to be given before the transition stage of labor. Talk to your medical team about what's appropriate. Often, during transition, a woman may feel as if she needs some sort of relief from the intensity of the pain to get her through, but at that point it's too close to the baby's arrival to administer medication safely. Fortunately, transition is pretty quick—keep reminding her of that.

HE SAYS:

Unfortunately, the drugs are available only for her.

QUESTIONS TO ASK

While your partner's in labor, there could be a lot going on that you might want to question. Go right ahead. It's your right to know what's going on and why.

Does she need to be induced? If pre-labor or early labor has gone on too long, or her water has broken but labor hasn't started, Pitocin (the synthetic form of oxytocin, the hormone that causes contractions) may be used to get contractions started. Once your partner is induced, she'll be attached to a fetal monitor, which will restrict her mobility and force her to labor on her back. Pitocin tends to amplify the intensity of labor and makes contractions more painful, so make sure pain medication is available for her if she wants it. Talk with your medical team about possible alternatives.

Does she need to be attached to a fetal and contraction monitor? If she's hooked up to a fetal monitor, she'll need to stay in one position so that the band around her belly, which is monitoring the baby, stays in place. This can be extremely uncomfortable and also frustrating if she wants to try different positions or move around. An internal fetal monitor, which is inserted through the vagina and attached to the baby's scalp, will also impede your partner's ability to move around.

Can she get out of bed if she's hooked up to any machines?
Ask if she can be unhooked from the machines from time to time so she can get up and move around.

Does she need an IV? Often hospitals will automatically set up an IV when a laboring woman is admitted, in case she needs medication. It isn't always necessary, and it will inhibit movement. Ask if she can get a heparin lock (heplock) instead, which is a small tube connected to a catheter in her vein. Basically, it provides quick and easy access should she need an IV in the future.

HE SAYS:

> The fewer things she is hooked up to, the better the experience will be in general.

Can she get medication? Medication is usually administered after she reaches 4 centimeters, and depending on the length of labor, she might need more at a later point, too. Keep track of how she's feeling, and if she wants medication, be her advocate.

STAGE 2 LABOR

Many people think Stage 2 is just about pushing. But there's much more to it than that. At this point, contractions are moving the baby through the birth canal. Now that she's fully dilated, the contractions may let up a bit, giving the mom-to-be a little break (relatively speaking) and a chance to get a bit of rest. Just because she's at 10 centimeters doesn't mean she should start pushing. She should let the contractions do the work and not push until she *really* feels the need to. When she's ready to push, it's often a relief—it feels good to actually be able to do something.

What's happening to her body

The baby is moving through the birth canal and getting ready to meet the world. Contractions are no longer pushing against a closed cervix—now each one helps her body move the baby out. There are more breaks than during transition, giving her a chance to catch her breath, rest a bit, and rebuild energy for major pushing.

HE SAYS:

> Stage 2 labor? If you're not good at technical jargon, just call it "pushing."

What she's feeling

She may feel a second wind. Being able to actually do something, as in pushing, can give her a new sense of involvement and purpose. And she might feel as if she's found a little respite, as the time between contractions lengthens. For some women, much of the fear and anxiety turns to a sense of focus as birth is imminent. Other women can feel very vulnerable, scared, and emotional during this final part.

What you can do

- Help her find a comfortable position. Eventually she'll find something that is the right fit.

- Help her breathe through each contraction. As she pushes, encourage her to breathe out—and not to hold her breath. This part is all about opening up and letting things out.

- She may grunt, groan, scream, or curse. It's all good—support whatever it is she needs to do.

- When the baby crowns (his/her head becomes visible), ask if she wants to touch it. This can be a powerful motivator. Feeling the baby's head lets her know the ordeal is almost over.

- Suggest she look in a mirror to see the baby crown, but if she says no, that's okay. It's not for everyone.

- Remember, you don't have to watch, either. If you're squeamish, stay up by her head and watch from her vantage point.

- Keep reminding her the baby's almost here. Every push, every contraction, brings him or her closer.

- When the baby's finally born, enjoy the moment with her! No matter how she got here—natural, Cesarean, with or without meds—seeing the baby for the first time is a joy. Savor it. Revel in it.

- Make sure the baby is brought to her at the earliest possible moment.

- Take photos!

- After the baby arrives, don't forget the new mom and her feelings. It's easy for everyone to get caught up in the excitement of a new baby, but the mom just went through one of the most emotional, not to mention physically draining, experiences of her life.

HE SAYS:

> Thank god, it's over. You did it! Okay, enough self-congratulation. Make sure mother and baby are getting quality bonding time. And take a turn yourself. It's okay to wait until after things get cleaned up.

BACK LABOR

Back labor is when the baby is turned so its back rests against the mother's spine—normally, the baby's front is against her spine. When this occurs, contractions can be much more painful than usual. Have your partner change positions often, until she finds something bearable. Being on her hands and knees is often the most comfortable. While she's in that position, encourage her to rock her pelvis from side to side. Ice or heat packs might alleviate her discomfort somewhat. Firm pressure on her back could help, as well. Make sure she's not lying on her back—that exacerbates the problem.

HE SAYS:

Don't let her lie flat on her back, even if it's the preference of the medical staff.

STAGE 3 LABOR

After the baby arrives, the placenta has to be delivered. This can take up to 30 minutes or so after the baby's birth.

HE SAYS:

This is by far the weirdest part, because nobody ever mentions it. You're like, what the hell is that thing?

What's happening to her body

She'll still be having contractions, but they'll be mild, almost like menstrual cramps. During this time, the medical staff will check for tears and do any stitching that's necessary. The umbilical cord needs to be cut—if you're so inclined, you might ask to cut it yourself. The baby is still getting oxygen through the cord, so it shouldn't be cut until it stops pulsating.

HE SAYS:

Don't be nervous about cutting the cord, although if you see it pulsating, I would run. In any event, don't worry—your snipping technique will have no bearing on whether the baby will have an innie or an outtie.

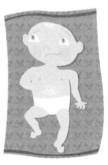

What she's feeling

It's impossible to predict how a new mom will feel after childbirth. Emotions run the gamut from elation, joy, and relief to exhaustion, disappointment, and fear—and everything in between. One whole chapter of her life, where she was the center of attention, is over. Her world has changed forever. It's hard to believe that she might be depressed, given the joyous occasion of having a baby. Keep in mind that she's likely to be exhausted and is facing a huge life change. Be patient with her if she's feeling low after the birth. If her dark mood persists, though, by all means seek out professional help.

HE SAYS:

You can be pretty sure that you're not going to be the center of attention at home either. Keep yourself relevant: learn how to change a diaper.

What you can do

- Tell her that you love her and are proud of her.

- If the baby needs any special care, go with him.

- Make sure the new mom and baby get to spend time bonding. If the hospital staff wants to separate them before they're ready, see if you can buy them some more time together. In instances when the baby needs to be taken away, ask to have her brought back to Mom as soon as possible.

- Make sure your partner gets any assistance she needs for breastfeeding. There are often lactation consultants on staff at the hospital to help mother and baby get started.

- When she's ready, start sharing the news. It could be that she just wants it to be the three of you for a while. Honor her wishes. You can never get this time back.

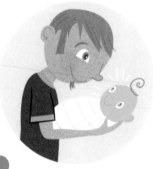

HE SAYS:

Photograph the new mom in these first moments with the baby. She will be forever grateful to you. Definitely get her permission, though, before you upload those pics of her looking like she's just been knocked out of an ultimate-fighting event.

BIRTHING OPTIONS

There are so many options for where and how to give birth. Some women choose to be at home, others at a birthing center, and still others in the hospital. Some want to give birth underwater, some want to be holding on to birthing bars, and others want to give birth with an epidural. Some want to have only their partner present, while others invite extended family to the event. Some women use an ob-gyn, while others choose a midwife practice. Regardless of where, how, and with whom a woman chooses to give birth, a wonderful option is to have a doula—someone who attends the birth as an extra support for the mother, baby, and family.

HE SAYS:

Elissa wanted a doula for our second child. I wasn't immediately comfortable with the idea of having a stranger at the birth, but she turned out to be a really great presence. Of course, we all met first and game-planned how we hoped the birth would go. And when things got out of control during transition, the doula locked eyes with Elissa and helped her calm down and focus. She helped us both have the birth experience we wanted.

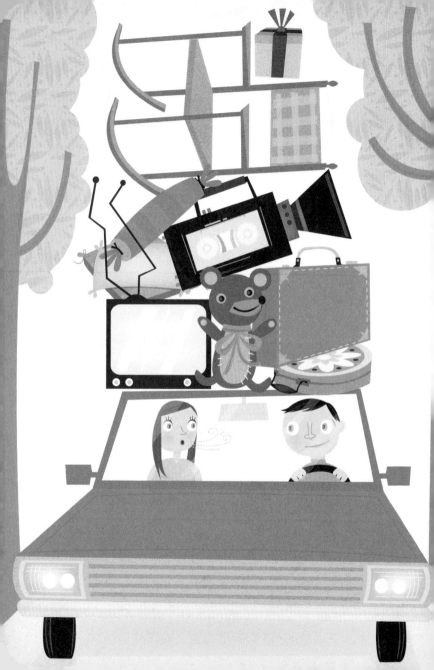

What to
BRING

If you're getting anywhere near the delivery date, you've probably already packed a hospital bag. And it probably contains mostly essentials for your partner and the baby. But you'll be there for the duration, too, and it's important that you're also taken care of. So here are some suggestions to make your hospital stay a little more comfortable, as well as a few ideas for things you can pack for her that she might not have thought about.

Keep in mind that this will hopefully be a short hospital stay, and that you'll be going home with a baby and all the additional stuff that goes along with that little person—like diapers, those great baby blankets they use at the hospital, an infant bathtub, plus the baby gifts that seem to start arriving almost at the moment of birth. Don't overpack. (Jon brought two giant suitcases to the hospital for my first birth—it looked like we were going to Bermuda for a week.)

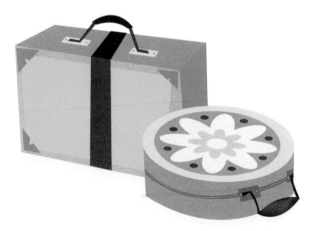

JUST FOR YOU

- *Sweats.* Throw an extra pair into your bag. You could be spending time with her on her bed, or kneeling or squatting on the floor. You'll be more comfortable in sweatpants.

- *Bathing suit.* It sounds crazy, but should your partner want to take a shower, and want you with her, the nursing staff will most likely appreciate that you're wearing some basic swimwear. Flip-flops are nice to have on hand, too.

- *Change of clothes.* Whether her labor lasts 8 hours or 48 hours, you'll be happy to have something clean to change into when it's over.

- *Snacks.* Throw some energy bars into your bag. Hospital cafeterias provide marginal fare, at best. Plus, disappearing to grab a quick bite and then getting stuck on a cafeteria line won't endear you to your partner.

- *Cell phone and charger.* No, you shouldn't run down your battery by chatting while she's in labor, but you want to make sure that after the baby arrives you can call everyone you want to share the good news with. You don't want your phone to die halfway down the list.

- *Music equipment.* Remember, she's in charge of what gets played, but make sure she can play it. Bring the CDs and CD player, iPod, batteries, chargers, plugs—

whatever you need to make sure you can play what she wants to hear.

- *Camera equipment.* Whatever you need—film, memory cartridges, chargers, video camera, etc.—make sure you've got it ready to go. Know that not all hospitals are okay with videotaping births. Not all partners are okay with videotaping births, either. Make sure you know what both the hospital and the mother-to-be will allow.

- *Phone list.* It's so exciting to let everyone know what's going on! Make sure you have all the numbers you need with you.

- *Toothbrush/mouthwash/breath mints.* Just imagine how you'll both feel after hours and hours in a stale hospital room, lots of deep breathing, not a lot of eating—do we need to say more?

- *Deodorant.* Bring some and keep reapplying. It will make the experience better for everyone.

- *Water.* Stick a couple of bottles in your bag.

- *Money.* Include lots of change for the hospital vending machines.

- *This book.* It'll help get you through every step of labor.

JUST FOR HER

- *Birth plan.* Bring a written list of your wishes and preferences for childbirth, and be ready to be her advocate in following it as much as possible.

- *Lemon slices.* Put some in a Ziploc bag and let her have a whiff if she feels sick to her stomach—the smell of lemon helps alleviate nausea.

- *Lollipops. LifeSavers. Hard candies.* When she's restricted to things she can suck on, it's nice to give her something with a little flavor to break up the monotony of ice chips.

- *Aromatherapy aids.* Drizzle some cotton balls with lavender or chamomile oil and put them in a Ziploc bag (if you bring both scents, make sure to keep them in separate bags). Inhaling either of these scents will help her relax. Make sure not to put the oil directly on her body—she may not like the smell, or may change her mind and want to get rid of it. Instead, put the oil on something, like a washcloth, that can be removed from the room if the scent bothers her. Or mix a few drops of essential oil with distilled water in a misting bottle, so you can lightly spray it around the room.

- *Small plastic bags.* Stick some in your pockets. Really. Should she be nauseated on the way to the hospital, she can throw up in a bag and you can throw it away. Much better there than all over the backseat of your car.

- *Toothbrush/mouthwash/breath mints.* See facing page.

- *Flowers.* **If you can pick some up on the way, great—or else buy some at the hospital gift shop. Flowers make a terrific focal point during labor.**

- *Snacks.* **After the baby arrives, your partner might be starving. She just worked really, really hard, and if it's the middle of the night, there may not be anyplace that's open and serving food. Having something on hand for her to chow down on—energy bars, nuts, and dried fruit are good choices—will keep you both happy.**

- *Photos.* **Photos are a lovely reminder of loved ones. Have her choose a few to bring along, and prop them up where she can see them. Personal items in her room will make her feel a little more grounded.**

- *Moisturizer/lip balm.* **With all the breathing, she'll need it.**

- *Presents.* **What if you brought a little present for the baby, hidden in your bag? Your thoughtfulness will be remembered for years to come. A little gift for your partner would be lovely, too.**

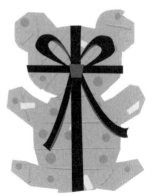

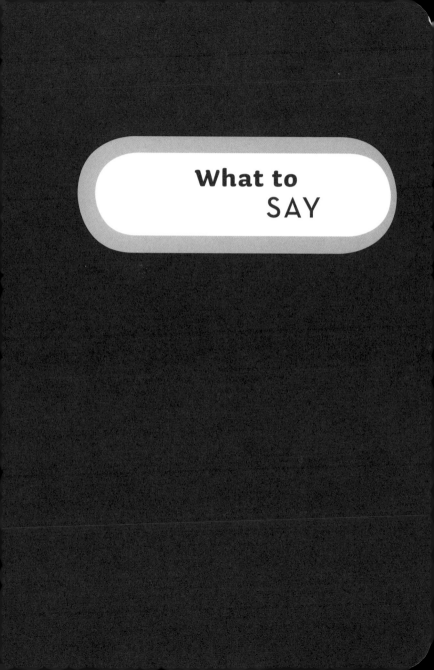

What to
SAY

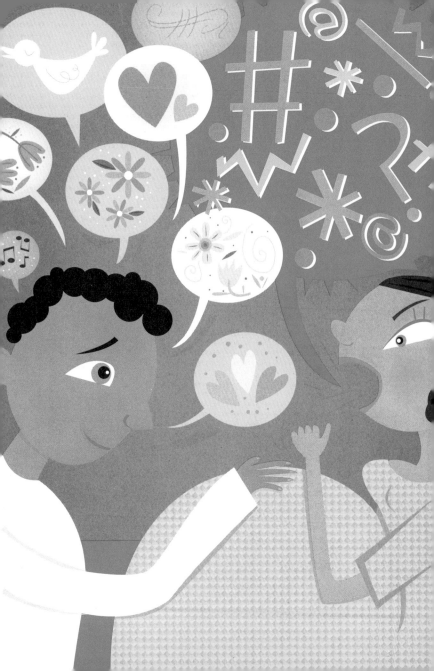

Words of comfort can make all the difference in the world when things get scary, intense, painful, and emotional. And labor can certainly be all of these things at one time. Here you'll find soothing words to share with your partner, to help her visualize herself in a more peaceful place, or to help her imagine her body relaxing and opening for the baby.

You can skip around, try them all out, or stick to just one phrase that's working. You'll find prompts to help her concentrate on her breathing, and visualization ideas to get her mind into a more relaxed and open place. Staying calm and positive will help keep her anxiety and fear from taking over. Remind her that whatever she's going through is only temporary and will eventually end. While it might feel like she'll be in labor forever, that's not physically possible.

HE SAYS:

Women in labor can say some crazy things that wouldn't usually come out of their mouths. Totally normal. If she goes off the deep end, lock eyes with her, move in close, and talk her back down.

While we can't stress enough that encouraging and supportive words are important for a laboring woman to hear, remember, of course, that at times she might tell you to shut up, scream at you, glare at you like you're the enemy, blame you, curse at you, or hate you. And that's just fine. She's going through an experience you can't imagine. Hard, scary, and/or frustrating as it might be, don't get caught up in it; just let it roll off you and be there for her. Look deep into her eyes and give encouragement, under-standing, empathy, and empowerment. Even if it seems that she's turning to the dark side, use the following words to bring her back to a better place.

HE SAYS:

If you feel funny about or uncomfortable with the following affirmations, you'll probably do better working with the breathing prompts. The way your partner is breathing and the quality of her breath are easy to track and be aware of. You can also breath along with her, which is a good way to stay connected.

TO EMPOWER

- You are beautiful.
- You can do this.
- You are so strong.
- You are powerful.
- This baby is so lucky to have you as its mother.
- You should be so proud of yourself.

- You are amazing.

- I always knew you could do this.

- Your hair looks great.

HE SAYS:

> So what if that last one's a lie? There's only going to be one mirror in the room, and it's not going to be pointed at her face (it's for her to watch the baby's birth).

TO COMBAT ANXIETY

- You're doing great.

- You can handle this.

- Believe that you can do this.

- Your body is designed to give birth.

- This is all so the baby can get to us.

- It's okay if it hurts.

- Let go of your fear.

- Everything is fine.

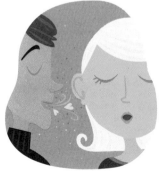

WHAT TO SAY

TO PROMOTE CONCENTRATION

- Trust your body, it knows what to do.
- Focus on a smooth, easy birth.
- Concentrate on the baby coming.
- Imagine your body opening up to let the baby through.
- Every contraction brings us closer to meeting the baby.

TO CONNECT THE TWO OF YOU

- I am so proud of you.
- You are my hero.
- Hang in there.
- I love you.
- Squeeze my hand if you need to.
- I can't believe our mothers did this.
- I can see how hard you're working.
- You are doing such a good job.
- I can't even imagine how this feels.
  (No, you can't.)

TO COMBAT DESPAIR

These affirmations are great at the very end, when she feels ready to give up but she's so close to meeting the baby.

- I can't wait for us to meet the baby.
- This is the hardest part.
- This is only temporary.
- I know this feels endless, but it won't last forever.
- The baby is coming.
- You are not alone. I'm here for you.

TO RELAX

Relaxing during labor? It's all relative. Helping her relax during childbirth means letting her body do what it knows how to do and keeping her mind from adding anxiety and fear. If you can keep her calm and focused, her body will do the work of birthing. Breathing prompts and visualizations are super-helpful here. Try these relaxing phrases, too.

- Let the contraction wash over you.
- Feel your body opening like a flower.
- *(After a contraction)* Take a deep breath and let that contraction go.

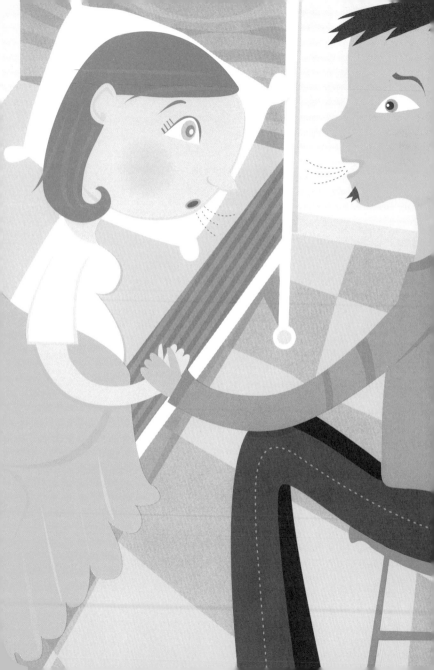

BREATHING PROMPTS

Breathing is fundamental during childbirth. Okay, breathing is fundamental all the time—but during labor, concentrating on it is essential. Deep, controlled breathing is an effective way to help relieve stress, anxiety, and muscle tightness. If you can get your partner concentrating on her breathing, it means she won't be obsessing about contractions or dilating or discomfort. Focusing on breathing gives her a sense of calm and control. Plus, this is a great way for you to help. Give her prompts. Count out loud for inhales and exhales. Remind her not to hold her breath (women tend to do this, especially when pushing). And breathe with her—sometimes just watching you slowly breathe in and out will keep her on track.

Tell her:

- Breathe in through your nose, breathe out through your mouth.

- Breathe in . . . breathe out . . . breathe in . . . breathe out . . .

- Breathe in calm; breathe out tension.

- Breathe into the contraction.

- Fill your belly like it's a beautiful balloon.

- Breathe oxygen for the baby.

- Concentrate on your breath.

- Each breath brings the baby closer to meeting us.

- Slow your breathing down.

- Watch my breath and breathe with me.

- Breathe in through your belly button. Breathe out through your bottom.

- Let your breath move the baby.

- Breathe in for four. *(Count out loud: One, two, three, four.)*

  Hold it for a second.

  Now breathe out for four. *(Count out loud: One, two, three, four.)*

  Hold it for a second.

  Let's do it again.

HE SAYS:

Helping her concentrate on breathing is great for calming yourself down, too. Just remember, with all that heavy breathing: breath mints.

VISUALIZATIONS

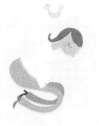

Visualization is a powerful tool to try during labor—helping your partner to imagine herself in a peaceful, calm place can make a tremendous difference for her. It's great to talk through some visualization ideas together before labor starts, so you have a sense of what kind of images work best for her. But it's hard for anyone not to relax when thinking about the beach (leave out the sand-in-the-bathing-suit part) or a beautiful sunset. Try some of these simple ideas as a starting point, and use your imagination and/or memories to bring your partner even further into the picture. You'll also find visualizations specifically meant to help her "see inside," open up, and make space for the baby.

HE SAYS:

Visualizations are a great thing, as long as your partner is in a receptive state to hear them. They aren't meant to alleviate acute anxiety, but to extend and deepen a sense of calm. Reading imagery about waterfalls to an acutely anxious woman is done at one's own risk. It helps to bring a vacation photo or two, to inspire you with words she'll relate to.

Beach

Imagine lying on the beach. Feel the sand supporting you.

The sun is warm on your skin.

Listen to the water gently lapping at the shore.

Imagine the waves, slowly rolling in and out.

There's a breeze moving the clouds slowly across the sky.

You are so comfortable here. It is calm and peaceful and beautiful.

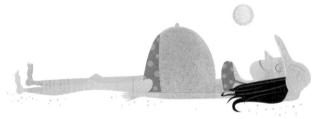

Waterfall

Imagine being next to a cascading waterfall.

Listen to the water splashing against the rocks as it falls and in the stream below.

The sun is glistening in the drops of water.

The water is gently misting over you.

The water is endlessly flowing over the top.

You can feel the rhythm of the waterfall.

It's powerful and relaxing at the same time.

Sunset

Imagine you're watching a beautiful sunset.

The sky is blue and purple and orange and pink.

The clouds seem to be lit from behind; their edges glow with pink and coral. The sun is deep orange.

It seems to shimmer as it dips lower and lower in the sky.

For a moment, all movement seems to stop right before the sun disappears.

The vibrant colors of sunset slowly fade as the sun falls below the horizon.

Stars appear as the sky deepens to dark blue.

You feel the warmth of the evening sky wrap around you.

The day is over. All is peaceful and quiet and calm.

Clouds

Imagine you are sitting on a cloud.

It feels like you are surrounded by soft silk.

Or suspended in a giant, fluffy cotton ball.

You sway slightly, as if you were suspended in a hammock.

Your body floats as if it were in water. You are weightless.

You float gently along, feeling peace and ease wash over you.

Everything is calm and quiet.

River

A flowing river is a good analogy for the feeling of labor—the experience of childbirth should just wash over her. The mom-to-be shouldn't get in the way of the moving current (contractions). Very conceptual, but it helps. At least try it.

Imagine a gently flowing river.

You can't see where it started. You can't see its end.

You're just watching the water slowly gliding by.

The water is lapping at the river's banks.

You can hear it softly lapping against the shore.

The sun is glinting across the water's surface.

The current is smooth and steady.

Small ripples appear on the surface every now and then.

You feel at ease and peaceful, at one with the river.

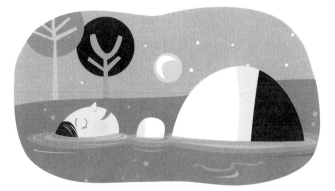

Flower

Visualizing opening and expanding is great for your partner —it helps her relax and open up for the baby.

Imagine you're looking at a rosebud.

Its petals are warm red; the color gets deeper at the edges.

The petals feel like soft velvet.

There are tiny water drops clinging to the leaves and stem.

Slowly, slowly, you can see it bloom.

The petals widen and expand. They soften.

You can smell the rose's sweet scent.

Now you can see deep inside the flower.

It is full of grace and beauty.

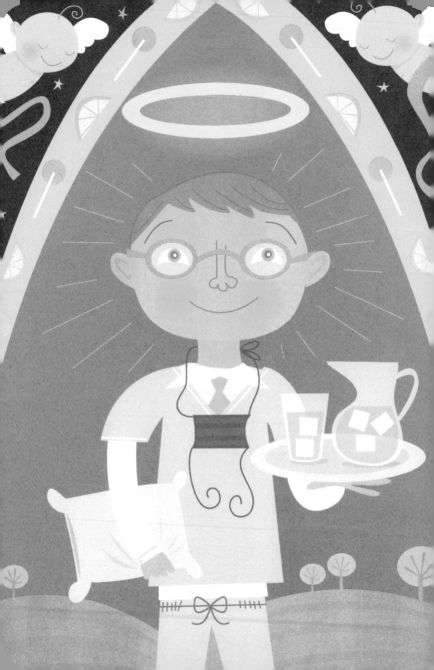

How to
COMFORT

Labor is hard work, and truly, there are times when, no matter what anyone does, your partner's not going to be comfortable. But there's plenty you can do to make a difference. Most important, stay close by, follow her lead, and be yourself (as long as you don't irritate her).

To make her feel calmer and more comfortable, remember these basics:

- *Be patient.* It may seem like forever, but the baby will eventually arrive. Truly.

- *Be present.* Stay close to her. Feeling you near will often be enough.

- *Be positive.* There will be times that she will be scared, feel hopeless, or want to give up. And sometimes things do get scary, crazy, or out of control. Regardless of what you're feeling inside, keep her spirits up.

- *Be thoughtful.* Stroke her cheek. Kiss her forehead. Show her that you love her and are proud of her. Little gestures can make a world of difference.

- *Be adaptable.* You may think you've found the answer to making her feel more comfortable. Maybe you remember something from your birthing class that you truly think will help, but she's not interested. Let it go. Great as they may be, don't force your ideas on her. Just try something else.

Also know that during labor, things can change at the drop of a hat. You have to be flexible. Everything you two talked about can get thrown out the window. If she wants medication, support her. If there needs to be some sort of intervention, let it happen. In the end, it's all about keeping the mom and baby safe and healthy.

- *Be the bigger person.* She may curse, scream, yell, and blame you for everything that she's going through. Truly, it can get ugly at times. But let it go. And don't take it personally.

HE SAYS:

> The challenge is that even if you're not naturally thoughtful, sensitive, or in tune with your partner's emotions and needs (and let's face it, how many of us are?), you need to get into the zone, because that's what the game is about. When in doubt, keep your mouth closed. What's most important is to be there, holding her hand or stroking her forehead. This kind of physical attention generally doesn't backfire.

CREATE A CALM SPACE

There are few places more stressful than a hospital—harsh lights, monitors beeping all the time, people coming in and out of your room at all hours, unpleasant colors, antiseptic smells. While many places now have birthing rooms that are supposed to look and feel less hospital-ish, there's still plenty you can do to help create a calm and soothing environment to help your partner feel more relaxed. No, you don't have to arrive at the hospital with an interior-design team, but you can easily do the following (a little advance preparation may be required).

Dim the lights.

Lower the shades, and turn off as many lights as you can. Bright lights can exacerbate tension.

Play music.

Have a collection of favorite CDs or a birth playlist good to go. Remember to bring something to play music on (CD player, iPod, etc.), and extra batteries or a cord to plug it in with.

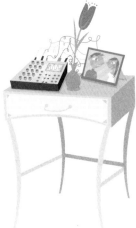

Don't rely on the hospital's audio equipment—the CD player in our delivery room didn't work. And if someone tells you that you can't use an electrical outlet, they probably don't want to listen to your music. Persist.

Use aromatherapy.

Soothing scents can bring a sense of calm to a chaotic situation. Suggest that your partner inhale a calming scent (see page 51) when she needs to relax a bit. Or grab that misting bottle and spritz around the room. Yes, real men can spritz—just make sure you don't spray her in the face.

Another thing to try: peel a grapefruit. Don't let her eat it (the acid in citrus fruits isn't good for her right now), but the scent of fresh grapefruit is cleansing and refreshing. Unless you put citrus fruit on your packing list, this is more likely something you'd do at home, not at the hospital.

HE SAYS:

If essential oils are beyond you, you can probably find some nice-smelling hand cream at a drugstore. Personally, I would leave this up to her—choosing the wrong scent can have consequences.

Bring photos and more.

Photos can make a hospital room feel more like home. If there are any special cards, small pieces of art, or drawings that you know would make her smile, throw those in the hospital bag, too.

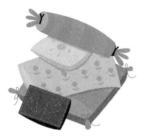

Pack pillows and blankets.

Does she have a favorite pillow? Small blanket? Teddy bear? Bring them. It may seem like you're packing for an extended cruise, but sometimes having something familiar close by can be incredibly comforting.

HE SAYS:

While you want to discuss what she wants to bring, make sure you sneak in a few items without telling her, too. It'll score you some major points for thoughtfulness.

Protect her privacy.

Turn off the phone (cell phones, too). Close the door. This shouldn't be an open-house party—unless she wants it to be, and that's pretty unlikely.

MAKE HER EVEN MORE COMFORTABLE

In addition, the following may help when soothing her requires a little something extra.

An extra layer

Warm socks. An extra sweater that zips or buttons up the front (a pullover-style sweater can be really hard to get on and off). Her own nightgown or a big T-shirt (she won't be particularly comfortable if her butt is sticking out of the hospital gown). A favorite blanket (depending on the room, the season, and her internal temperature, she could get hot or cold pretty quickly—hospital blankets just don't cut it).

Pillows

For those times when she wants to be in a bed, a pillow tucked under her knees or behind her back can feel really good.

Cold washcloths

Labor is really hard work, especially the pushing part. A cold washcloth on her forehead can bring welcome relief from all the sweating. At the back of her neck and under her arms can feel really wonderful, too.

Water, water, and more water

It is so important to stay hydrated during labor. You can offer her sips of water between contractions. Even if she only moistens her mouth, every little bit helps. And here's a great tip: use bendy straws. Just bend the straw toward her and she won't have to move her head.

Grape juice is great, too—lots of calories—and raspberry tea with honey is soothing and can help keep her energy up. Remember, if you're at the hospital, they may allow only ice chips so that her stomach is empty in the rare event that anesthesia is needed.

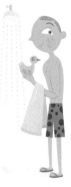

HE SAYS:

> Don't go overboard with the ice chips. She can use them as projectiles.

Even more water!

Suggest a shower. The warmth of the water, along with the sensation of water beating down on her, can be extraordinarily soothing and relaxing. Should she be up for it, feel free to join her. Just make sure to wear a bathing suit—you don't want to surprise the nurses. But if changing and moving into a shower is too much for her to handle, let it go and try something else.

Lip balm

All that work and heavy breathing can dry out her lips, which can be really uncomfortable. Have some lip balm ready (carry several, in different pockets) for her to re-moisturize her lips with.

Fresh lemon slices

If she's suffering from nausea, the scent of fresh lemons really helps. Have a Ziploc bag ready to pull out for her to sniff if she feels sick to her stomach.

Massage

Can you imagine how good a foot massage might feel when she's working hard during labor? Try it. A shoulder or back massage is great, too—even rubbing her temples helps to ease tension. Use slow, firm, gentle pressure (rubbing too fast can be really aggravating) and check out the following pages for ideas and techniques. Another idea: tennis balls in a sock. Really. Put three tennis balls in a sock, tie the open end shut, and then roll the whole thing across her back.

HE SAYS:

Tickling her feet is definitely not a good idea.

- *Seated massage.* Have her sit and lean forward, letting her head and arms rest on a flat surface in front of her (with pillows keeping her comfortable). Stand behind her and massage her shoulders and neck—places that typically hold a lot of tension. Then, using your thumbs, or the heels of your hands, massage her lower back—start at her sacrum (the bottom of the spine) and move up.

- *Side lying massage.* Have her lie on her side with one pillow under her head and another between her knees (if that's comfortable), and massage her lower back.

- *Temple massage.* Using your fingertips, rub her temples in a gentle circular motion.

Acupressure

This may sound a little farfetched, but give it a whirl. Acupressure uses finger pressure on specific points on the body for pain relief. Try holding one of 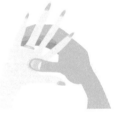 the following pressure points for a count of 6 to 10, then repeat 6 to 10 times. All three of these points are tender spots. Ask her when you've got it—she'll know if you're there or not. And don't be thrown by the technical terms these specific points are known by; you won't need to find her liver or spleen to put the pressure on.

1. The fleshy area between the thumb and forefinger (large intestine 4)

2. A spot about two inches above her inner ankle (spleen 6)

3. The spot between the big toe and second toe, on top of the foot (liver 3)

HE SAYS:

> I used pressure point No. 1 during Elissa's labor, and it really seemed to work! If only the Vulcan nerve pinch could be used instead of an epidural.

CHANGE POSITIONS

It's so important to change positions during labor. Staying in one place too long can get really uncomfortable. And remember, the typical labor scene you've seen on TV or in the movies, with the woman lying on her back in bed, is a terrible scenario in the real world.

HE SAYS:

> This can't be emphasized enough. The medical staff may want her on her back. In our first birth, the fetal monitor worked better when Elissa was on her back, so they insisted, but this made the pain excruciating, highlighting the importance of trying different positions!

Walking, as long as she's comfortable with it, is great for her. When she's upright, gravity helps keep the baby in the proper position, and the back-and-forth swaying of the hips helps move the baby along. Slow dancing is another option. Play music with a good mellow groove, hold her loosely, and do the junior high back-and-forth dance. This is a good way to help during contractions, as she can just lean into you.

Dancing may seem like a crazy idea, but gravity is a great asset during childbirth. If you can keep her upright, it will speed things along and should lessen her discomfort.

More position suggestions:

Squatting

While this is a great position to be in (it opens up the pelvis and lets gravity pull the baby down), it's hard to hold unless she's been practicing throughout pregnancy. Many hospitals have a squat bar, which helps by giving her something to hold on to.

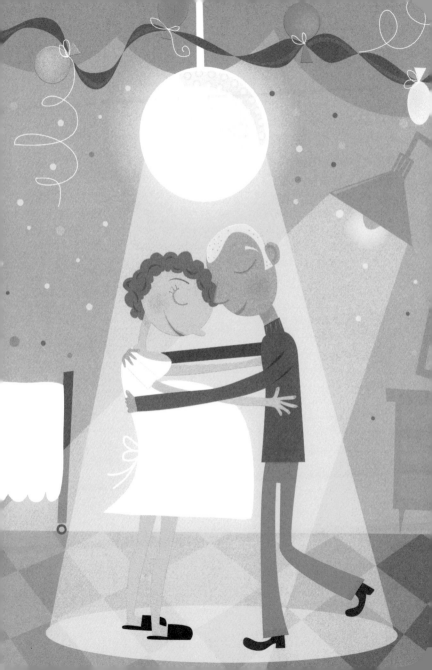

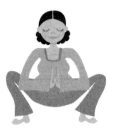

Elissa practiced squatting every day, and I challenged myself to keep up with her. I found out that my pelvis was not ready for childbirth (duh!). Nevertheless, our strength and flexibility increased dramatically in a very short period of time practicing. This, along with Kegels, is an exercise that I would really encourage in the lead-up to labor. The better shape she's in for the birth, the faster and better she'll snap back after.

On a birth ball

A birth ball (a.k.a. Pilates ball) is a nice thing to labor with. It moves with her, is supportive, and never gets tired. She can . . .

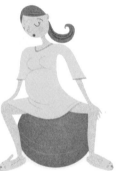

- *Sit on it.* She can sway back and forth, lean forward for support, gently bounce up and down.

- *Kneel into it.* Have her get on her knees and drape her chest over the birth ball. She can rest her face on her hands. This takes all pressure off her back and can be easier on her than just being on hands and knees.

- *Stand and lean into it.*

Personally, if there's a ball in the room, I'm going to be playing with it. Although it has the potential to amuse you during a long labor, it also has the potential to get you into trouble.

Lying on her side

This is a nice position when she needs a little rest. It gives her legs a break and keeps her off her back. Believe it or not, she might even be able to fall asleep between contractions.

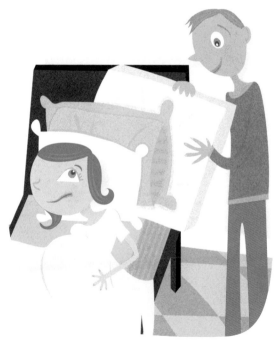

Leaning against you

This is a great position for both of you (and for the nurses, as you'll be out of their way). Climb up on her bed, lean against the headrest, and have her lean back against you, between your legs. The bonus is that you get to see just what she's seeing—as close a view as you'll ever have of giving birth. A tip: leave the jeans at home—sweats are far more comfortable.

HE SAYS:

Being on the bed also gives you easier access to the television remote and the up and down functions of the hospital bed, which, besides being fun to play with, are helpful for easing her discomfort.

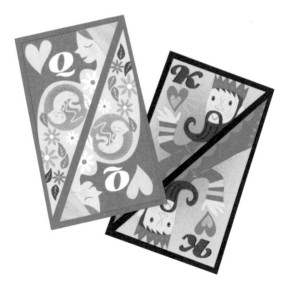

DISTRACT HER . . .

In early labor, distractions certainly have their place, especially when things are moving slowly. Suggest some of the following—she may be happy to have something else to think about.

Have a snack.

It's important that she keep her energy up. She doesn't need a steak dinner at this point, but something like dried fruit is full of calories that she'll need later. Ice pops are great—they're good for hydrating. Even the soothing sensation of licking a lollipop can make her happy for a bit.

HE SAYS:

Don't forget to get yourself something—you've got to eat too, right? Don't get anything too crunchy, anything that will leave residue on your fingers (no Cheetos!), or anything that she can smell—she's likely to be really cranky because you left her, even if she was the one who asked you to get food.

Play a game.

You don't need to start a game of Monopoly, but sometimes a simple card game—one that you can leave and come back to—can be a good way to pass time.

Watch TV.

Classic reruns can feel like comfort food. Or a favorite movie can relax and distract you both.

TAKE CHARGE

Be her advocate.

A woman in labor has enough to concentrate on, and as labor progresses, her attention moves more and more inward. Step up and take charge when the situation needs it.

Maintain calm and quiet around her.

Keep relatives away if she wants them away. Respect her wishes about that—remember, this is about her, not you or them. And remember, it's not mandatory to have lots of hospital personnel bustling in and out of the room. Ask them to stay out unless absolutely necessary.

HE SAYS:

It's okay to ban the medical residents from watching your partner give birth.

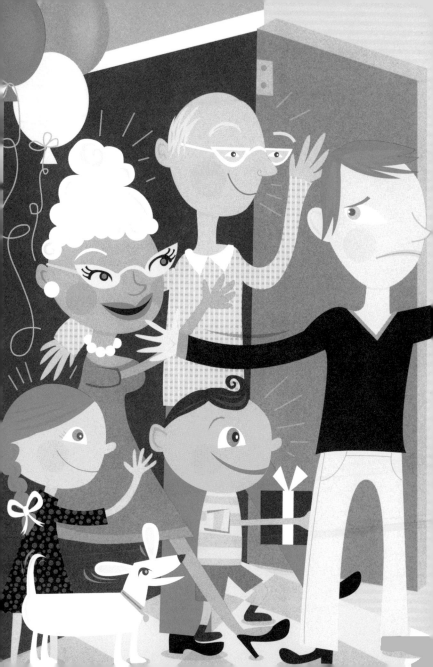

Know the birth plan.

It's important that you know and respect her wishes for this birth, and, if necessary, communicate them to the medical staff. Remember, it's her body and her childbirth, and while her choices might not be the same as yours, you're not the one pushing the baby out.

HE SAYS:

> Be polite, but let the staff know you mean business about keeping to the birth plan. Unless it's an important medical issue, stand your ground.

Be her focus.

When she hits really rough patches (especially around the transition stage, when she's fully dilated and getting ready to push), really take charge. Tell her to open her eyes, look straight into yours, and breathe with you. Keep her engaged in a focused connection.

Get her what she needs.

If it's pain medication, track down the doctor if you have to. If it's water to drink, or a lollipop to lick, go get it. She can't get these things for herself, so make yourself available.

Keep her posted.

Especially in the later stages of labor, when her focus turns inward, let her know what's going on. While everyone wants labor to go smoothly, there are times when it can get a little crazy. Ask the questions you need to, get her the help she needs, and stay positive for her.

Take care of yourself.

It's important for you to be at your best, and that's not easy if you're tired and hungry. Eat. Rest when you can. Put on deodorant. Change your shirt if that will make you feel better. And don't forget to pee.

HE SAYS:

Now you're talking.

FINAL THOUGHTS

In the end, there are three things, above all else, that will help you to help her through. Remember these and you'll be just what she needs you to be.

1. Follow her cues. Listen to what she says, and respond to how she's acting.

2. Always be close by.

3. Love her.

What Not to
DO, SAY, or BRING

For the most part, this book has focused on all the things you *should* do— comfort her, encourage her, etc. But what about the things you definitely should *not* do? I'm here to tell you that there are quite a few. Believe me, it's better to hear this from me than her. And it's better to hear it before the birth than after. Because even if you've done everything else right—down to feeding her ice chips at three-minute intervals—in her state, she's going to remember only the one idiotic thing you did by mistake.

Since labor can go on for a long time, it might not seem particularly out of the question to run out for some lunch. How bad could it be to pull out that brand-new issue of *Sports Illustrated*? Think again. What's tricky here is that something you wouldn't think twice about doing under ordinary circumstances will be remembered as appalling if you do it during labor. No one wants to be the guy that's remembered for taking a call from his stockbroker while his wife was in labor.

To help you avoid a number of bad moves, I conducted a poll to compile this list of don'ts. If none of the following faux pas, taken from real birth stories, sound like anything that could ever happen to you, that's great. But if you can see yourself possibly going down the same path, pay close attention.

DON'TS

- Don't chat on your cell phone with your friends.

- Don't return work calls.

- No checking your stocks, surfing on the wireless, or checking your e-mail.

- Blowing bubbles and chewing gum is generally not a great idea.

- You may have had a really long, hard day, but let her have the bed.

- Don't fight her for control of the remote—make sure you TiVo all important ballgames at least 48 hours in advance as you come down the stretch to the due date.

- Reading a newspaper is a bad idea in general, even if you give her first choice of the sections.

- Don't flirt with the nurses.

- Don't take inappropriate photos—you're not making a documentary for the National Geographic Channel. Remember, anything you shoot should have a "PG" rating.

- Don't let your mother or other relatives into the room or within earshot, unless your partner is *totally* fine with it.

- Don't socialize too much with the labor partner in the next delivery room.

- Don't mention the successes of other laboring women on the floor—that's *not* going to inspire her.

- Don't ask the doctor to bring you coffee.

- Cool as it is to watch, don't pay more attention to the contraction monitor than to her.

- Avoid the subject of personal-injury law when conversing with the medical staff.

- Don't pass out and need to be taken down to the emergency room to get stitches.

- Don't scatter your stuff around the delivery room and then ask her if she's seen your car keys.

- Don't discuss real estate or golf with the doctor while she's having contractions.

- Don't eat onions, garlic, or other obnoxious food, like Doritos or Cheetos.

- Don't tell her to go back to sleep if she wakes you up with contractions.

- Don't tell her that you heard it doesn't have to hurt.

- And, finally, whatever you do, don't do what I did—lie in her bed the morning after, eating her breakfast, while she packs the bags. Unfortunately, Elissa has the photo to prove it.

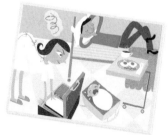

FILL IN THE BLANKS

Before labor begins, spend some time having the mom-to-be fill out the following lists. She may have very strong feelings about some categories, others, not at all. Could be when she's laboring, everything gets thrown out the window. But by thinking about her comfort in advance, you're working toward creating the kind of childbirth experience you are both hoping for.

I want to listen to . . .

- _____
- _____
- _____
- _____
- _____
- _____
- _____

To calm me down, I want you to say . . .

- _____
- _____
- _____
- _____
- _____
- _____

Don't ever say this . . .

- _____
- _____
- _____
- _____
- _____
- _____

I want you to ask the medical staff these questions . . .

- _____
- _____
- _____
- _____
- _____
- _____
- _____
- _____
- _____
- _____
- _____
- _____

FILL IN THE BLANKS

**These people are allowed
in the delivery room . . .**

- _____
- _____
- _____
- _____
- _____
- _____

**These people are *not* allowed
in the delivery room . . .**

- _____
- _____
- _____
- _____
- _____
- _____

**These are the people to call
after the baby is born . . .**

- _____
- _____
- _____
- _____
- _____
- _____
- _____
- _____
- _____
- _____
- _____
- _____
- _____

ACKNOWLEDGMENTS

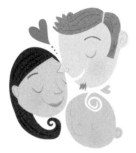

This project would not have been possible without the guidance from some remarkable women in the birthing community. There are not enough ways to say thank-you to Jessica Kramer, our doula at Jack's birth, for her knowledge, insight, and time. She brought, and continues to bring, awareness, light, and a sense of humor to everything. Thanks to Dr. Suzanne LaJoie, for bringing the same enthusiasm and support to this project that she brought to Jack's birth. Many thanks to Elaine Stillerman, LMT (www .MotherMassage.Net), for sharing her vast wealth of knowledge about childbirth, and to Ilana Stein at BirthFocus (www.birthfocus.com) and Lisa Spiegel at Soho Parenting (www.sohoparenting.com).

Thanks to all the mothers and fathers who shared their birth stories. Thanks to Jodi Warshaw, for giving us the opportunity to do this project. And thanks to Isabel and Jack, whose arrival into this world created the blueprint for this book.

RESOURCES

Bradley, Robert. *Husband-Coached Childbirth: The Bradley Method of Natural Childbirth*. New York: Bantam, 1996.

Dick-Read, Grantly. *Childbirth Without Fear: The Principles and Practice of Natural Childbirth*. London: Pinter & Martin Ltd, 2005.

Kennedy, Michelle. *It Worked for Me: 1001 Real-Life Pregnancy Tips*. New York: Barron's Educational Series, 2004.

Linden, Ann, C.N.M. "The Stages of Labor." July 2005. http://parentcenter.babycenter.com/refcap/177.html

Mikes, Beverly, M.D. "Stages of Labor—What to Expect During Childbirth." http://www.expectantmothersguide .com/library/philadelphia/EPHlabor.htm

Mongan, Marie. *HypnoBirthing: A Celebration of Life*. Concord, NH: Rivertree Hypnosis Institute, 1998.

Simkin, Penny. *The Birth Partner*, 2nd edition. Boston: Harvard Common Press, 2001.

Sears, Martha, and William Sears. *The Birth Book: Everything You Need to Know to Have a Safe and Satisfying Birth*. New York: Little, Brown, 1994.

Stillerman, Elaine. "Partner Labor Support Massage." *Massage Magazine*, November/December 2000.

"The Process of Labor: Pre-Labor vs. True Labor."
http://babies.sutterhealth.org/laboranddelivery/lab

Warnus, Susan. *Darn Good Advice: Pregnancy*. New York: Barron's Educational Series, 2005.

INDEX

Acupressure, 78–79

Affirmations, 56–59

Anxiety, combating, 57

Aromatherapy, 51, 73

Back labor, 41

Birth balls, 82–83

Birth plan, 51, 88

Braxton Hicks contractions, 19

Breastfeeding, 44

Breathing prompts, 61–62

Cesarean sections, 20

Charge, taking, 86, 88–89

Childbirth
  Cesarean sections, 20
  options for, 45
  unpredictability of, 11

Comforting
  basics of, 70–71
  techniques for, 72–90
  words for, 55–59

Concentration, promoting, 58

Contractions
  Braxton Hicks, 19
  in Stage 1, 26, 27–28, 29, 32
  in Stage 2, 38
  in Stage 3, 42

Despair, combating, 59

Distractions, 83–84

Doulas, 45

Due dates, 18

Epidural, 35

Fetal monitors, 36

Heparin lock, 37

Hospital, trip to
  packing for, 48–52
  timing of, 28

IVs, 37

Labor
  approaching, 18–20
  back, 41
  changing positions during, 79–84
  inducing, 36
  pre-, 21, 23
  Stage 1, 26–34
  Stage 2, 38–40
  Stage 3, 42–44

Lip balm, 77

Lists, 95–99

Massage, 77–78

Medication, 35, 37

Mistakes, 92–94

Mucous plug, 21

Music, 72–73

Packing, 48–52

Photographs, 44, 50, 52, 74

Pitocin, 36

Placenta, 42

Positions, changing, 79–84

Pre-labor, 21, 23

Relaxation, 59

Squatting, 80, 82

Supportive words, 55–59

Umbilical cord, cutting, 42

Visualizations, 63–67

Water, 76

Water breaking, 24